NATURAL
BEAUTY

NATURAL BEAUTY

MAKING AND USING PURE AND SIMPLE BEAUTY PRODUCTS

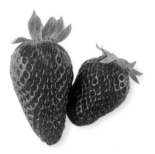

GAIL DUFF

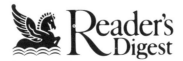

PUBLISHED BY THE READER'S DIGEST ASSOCIATION LIMITED
LONDON • NEW YORK • SYDNEY • CAPE TOWN • MONTREAL

A READER'S DIGEST BOOK

Published by
The Reader's Digest Association Limited
11 Westferry Circus
Canary Wharf
London E14 4HE

ISBN 0 276 42361 5

A CIP data record for this book is available from the British Library.

This book was designed and produced by
Breslich & Foss Ltd
20 Wells Mews
London W1 3FJ

Edited by Janet Ravenscroft
Designed by Roger Daniels
Illustrations by Lynette Conway

Printed in Hong Kong

CONTENTS

Foreword

Natural beauty is about feeling good on the inside so that you look good on the outside. It is about taking care of your whole being, and that means eating healthily and exercising, as well as looking after your skin and hair. It is not about putting on layers of make-up or being liberal with the hairspray, but about caring for yourself so that you look good without artificial embellishment. Of course, you can enhance the effect with make-up, but it is what is there naturally that makes the real difference.

The outside of your body is like a barometer. If you are happy and relaxed it shows, just as it shows if you are sad, tired or depressed, have eaten badly, drunk too much or not had enough exercise. So your lifestyle is the thing to work on first. Then you should take care of your outside by cleansing your body and by moisturising, nourishing, and when necessary, exfoliating your skin.

Making your own, or at least some of your own, beauty treatments is just part of this general care. Experimenting with lotions and potions is also highly rewarding and great fun. You might save a little money,

you will certainly know where your face, hair and body preparations come from and what they contain.

As I wrote this book, I was aware that no one in this day and age is going to be able to follow every beauty routine contained within it every day; there would be no time to do anything else. Use the treatments whenever you feel like pampering yourself or when you feel that a part of you needs special treatment, and gradually absorb the advice about general health and diet. Set aside certain days when you can experiment with things like creams and lotions. Get to know the quick and easy treatments that can be worked into your daily routine. Keep certain things like sun protection in the back of your mind at all times. Sneak in face or hand exercises whenever you have a moment. If you come to care more about yourself, how you feel and what you need, then I think I will have succeeded.

GAIL DUFF

BEAUTY FROM THE INSIDE

'Beauty is only skin deep' is an old cliché, but there is no better way of saying that the skin reflects whatever is going on inside your body. You can cover skin with moisturisers and make-up, but without feeding it well and caring for it from the inside you can rarely be truly beautiful.

Skin protects and supports the delicate tissues and vital organs that lie just beneath the surface. Our skin breathes and excretes waste materials and provides a growing pad for hair. It is fed nutrients and oxygen by tiny blood vessels that in turn pick up their cargoes from the food we take in and the air we breathe.

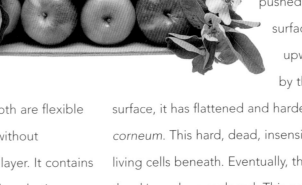

Skin is made up of two layers: the outer epidermis and the inner dermis. Both are flexible and elastic to allow movement of the body without distorting the skin. The dermis is the thicker layer. It contains blood vessels that bring nourishment and a lymphatic system that drains waste. Here also are two types of stretchy fibre, known as collagen fibres, that are made of protein and elastin. Collagen fibres give the skin the 'stretch-and-spring-back' quality that helps it to withstand bumps and knocks. Hairs begin their growth in the dermis, and nerve endings and hair follicles found here make the skin sensitive to touch and pain. Sweat glands in the dermis release moisture that

helps to control the body's temperature. Sebum, a natural lubricant and moisturiser, is produced in the sebaceous glands in the dermis. It mixes with sweat and forms a thin film on the skin called the acid mantle. This lends protection against infection and bacteria.

Skin cells are formed in what is called the *stratum germinativum* (the layer where growth begins). This is the lowest layer of the epidermis. The cells are continually replaced from beneath, so a new cell is gradually pushed upwards towards the surface. As the cell moves upwards it begins to die, and by the time it reaches the surface, it has flattened and hardened to form the *stratum corneum*. This hard, dead, insensitive layer protects the living cells beneath. Eventually, the old cells flake away from the skin and are replaced. This process is called desquamation and takes an average of twenty-one to twenty-eight days. The younger the skin, the quicker this cycle of renewal will be.

Skin is a vital, functioning part of us, yet how often is 'a lifestyle for a healthy skin' mentioned? There are 'healthy heart', 'stress reducing' and 'cancer preventive' lifestyles by the score, but skin seems to lose out.

Skin reflects the state of our body and our mind. Feeling run down? Then look in the mirror. Your skin will not look its sparkling best either. Have you eaten too much fast food? Then watch those spots appear in the more oily parts of your face. Have you been on a crash diet, eating nothing but lettuce leaves for days? Perhaps the skin on your arms or legs has gone dry and flaky. Does stress attack you in the middle of the night? Watch for the dark rings under your eyes. The better things are inside, the more naturally beautiful you will look.

GENERAL HEALTH

Health is a general state of well-being. To achieve it, take care of yourself: eat a balanced diet, drink alcohol in moderation, don't smoke, get enough sleep, try to reduce stress, and exercise as often as possible. Simple, really. Sounds boring? Well, try it and see. You will probably find that the healthier you feel, the more energy you have, and a person with a lot of energy very often has a greater capacity for enjoying life. If it sounds like an impossible lifestyle, make small changes first and see how things develop.

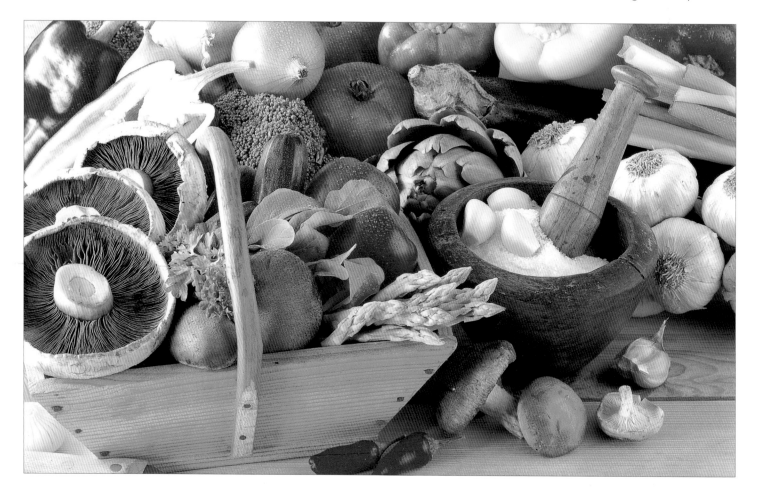

Breakfast:

Wholemeal toast with honey or unsweetened jam

Poached egg on wholemeal toast

Muesli or other wholemeal cereal with milk or plain yoghurt and chopped fruit

Fresh chopped fruit with plain yoghurt

Light meal:

Small piece of grilled or poached fish

Large mixed salad with small amount of protein-rich food

Wholemeal sandwiches with salad filling

Baked potato with a little butter or low-fat spread

Homemade or other nourishing vegetable soup with wholemeal bread

Homemade dip with vegetables

Fresh fruit for dessert

Main meal:

Small meat or vegetarian protein dish with potatoes, whole grain rice or pasta, and at least two other vegetables

Fruit salad with plain yoghurt for dessert

Snacks:

Fresh fruit

Fingers of raw vegetables

Wholemeal biscuits

Plain yoghurt

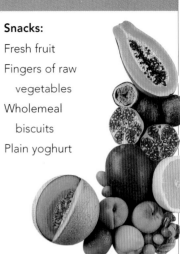

When you are young, you can get away with a bad diet, a hectic lifestyle and lack of sleep and still look great. But there will come a day when you look in the mirror and see the first grey hair or the first wrinkle. If you take extra care as early as possible, you may well be delaying the onset of those first signs of ageing.

DIET

A healthy diet should provide all the nutrients a body needs: protein for bodybuilding, carbohydrates for energy, fats in moderation for lubrication, a wide selection of vitamins and minerals for the proper functioning and repair of body tissues, plus fibre to help eliminate waste.

Eating a lot of any one food, however nourishing it is, will give you plenty of one or two nutrients and none of any of the others. A variety of foods eaten every day will provide a wide range of different nutrients. Try to include some carbohydrate foods, such as wholemeal bread, pasta and rice; at least four servings each of fresh fruit and vegetables; protein foods such as lean meat, fish, cheese, eggs, beans and nuts. Combine the last two with a whole grain food so you get the right kind of protein.

Some fat is necessary for good health, but you should keep the amount of animal fats you consume to a minimum. By all means have butter on your toast, but don't overdo it. Choose lean meat and cook it with sunflower or olive oil. In moderation, nuts are a good source of 'healthy' fat.

The fresher and less processed a food, the more nutrients it contains. If it has been chopped, cooked, mixed with other ingredients or dried, it will not contain the same goodness it began with. For optimum health, buy fresh ingredients and cook them yourself (or eat them raw).

Sugar is a highly refined carbohydrate that brings no nutrients with it in its white form, and an insignificant number when left brown. Too much sugar piles on the calories and also uses up essential B vitamins in its digestion. Try to cut it down.

Processing also includes the refinement of carbohydrate foods such as wheat or rice. When the whole grain of the wheat is ground to make wholemeal flour, the tiny bud (the germ) and the outer coating (the bran) are retained. The germ contains most of the nutrients. The bran provides the fibre that helps us to eliminate waste. If a body cannot eliminate waste, the skin may develop a sallow look. If you eat a balanced, relatively high-fibre diet, with plenty of raw fruits and vegetables, you should have no problems.

Extra bran used to be a recommended remedy, but bran alone can deplete the body's iron supplies. It is far better to eat a high-fibre cereal or wholewheat bread. High-fibre foods are also more satisfying and prevent us from overeating. Whenever possible, therefore, choose wholemeal bread and pasta, and brown rice. Other fibre-rich foods are fresh fruits and vegetables. Eat them whenever you can, as desserts, as part of a meal and as snacks between meals. They provide a wide range of vitamins and minerals and help ensure a healthy skin.

Water is essential for good health. It moisturises your skin from the inside and helps to flush waste and toxins from the body. Ideally you should drink eight glasses of water a day. If you find mineral water in this quantity too expensive, drink filtered tap water. Cut down on caffeine-rich drinks such as tea or coffee, choosing herb teas instead.

Dietary enemies

Both smoking cigarettes and drinking alcohol deplete the body's vitamin supply, especially of vitamins B and C, which are essential for maintaining a healthy skin. Toxins from alcohol and cigarette smoke are carried around the body in the bloodstream and smoking can restrict the blood flow to the skin. Coarse, ageing skin can be the result.

Many medications, such as antibiotics, can upset the skin's natural flora. This is because our skin is home to friendly bacteria that help to combat germs. Antibiotics are not choosy. They may kill off harmful bacteria, but they also kill off the ones we need, both in the digestive system and in the skin. If you are on prescribed medicines, the simple remedy is to eat at least 150 ml (5 fl oz) plain yoghurt every day while the course of treatment lasts and for two weeks thereafter.

SLEEP

Getting plenty of sleep is one of the other major contributors to maintaining healthy and glowing skin. During sleep, the body can repair itself undisturbed. It can also begin the process of ridding the tissues of toxins and waste materials. Without sleep, skin can develop a lack of tone and begin to look rather loose and baggy. Too many late nights can lead to dark rings under the eyes and premature ageing of the skin.

The body naturally relaxes as you sleep. All tightness leaves the muscles and this, in turn, helps to smooth out expression-formed wrinkles in the face. Dreams, even though you may not remember them, can help you to sort out day-to-day problems, thus relieving you of stress the following day.

People differ in the amount of sleep that they need. By the time you are an adult you probably have a good idea of how much you need, even though you may not adhere to it. Average sleep needs are from six to eight hours, and the hours before midnight are the most valuable when it comes to restful sleep. The body responds best to the same pattern of sleep, week by week. If possible, make certain nights late nights and others early ones. Bodies like routine, even if people don't.

In order to sleep, both your mind and body should be relaxed. Some people can just get into bed and fall asleep right away; others, for a variety of reasons, have difficulty sleeping. Try as many of the following as possible:

• Stop working. You have put in a busy day; you deserve to rest. Whether it is ironing, washing up or doing office work, make a conscious decision to stop.

• You may think that watching the television or a video is one of the most relaxing things that you can do, but films and documentaries can stir your emotions. Turn off the set.

• Enjoy the silence or put on a relaxing tape. Don't let anyone else choose the tape for you.

• Make yourself a warm drink made from milk – which is rich in calcium and promotes sleep – or a herbal drink designed for bedtime. Avoid tea and coffee at bedtime.

• If possible, eat your main meal two hours before going to bed to allow it to digest and to get rid of any uncomfortable 'full' feeling. Don't eat anything rich just before bedtime, but don't go to bed hungry. Have something like plain crackers, wholemeal biscuits or a small sandwich about half an hour before you retire.

• If you have to remember something the next day, write it down and leave it in a prominent place outside the bedroom. The same applies to problems. Write them down and resolve to deal with them in the morning.

• Try to resolve household arguments before going to bed. If you are angry or upset, sleep may not come easily.

• Warm baths are relaxing last thing at night. Pamper yourself. Add some relaxing, perfumed bath preparation or/and light a candle instead of turning on the light. Lie back and let your tension float away.

• Keep your bedroom as neat as possible so that it is a special place you enjoy going to. Light some incense or vaporise some perfumed oil, choosing relaxing scents, not the stimulating ones. Put water into the top of a vaporiser and add a few drops of essential oil to it. Then burn a shallow candle or nightlight underneath. Electric vaporisers are also available.

• Choose candlelight instead of electric light. (Make sure to blow out the candles before falling asleep.)

• Make love with your partner. This may well keep you awake longer than you intended, but sleep is always quick to arrive and is very deep afterwards.

EXERCISE

Exercise is important because it brings extra oxygen into your system and increases blood circulation. This means there is a greater turnaround of nutrients and waste products in every organ of your body, including your skin and hair. Keeping your system cleansed and vital helps you feel and look good.

There are two types of exercise. One is active, such as a workout in the gym or a set of aerobic exercises. The other is more passive, such as yoga or other forms of stretching exercise, and concentrates on the body's suppleness. In an ideal world we would include each in our regular routine.

Aerobic exercise should make you slightly out of breath, but not leave you breathless and exhausted. You should exercise at least twenty minutes, three times a week, preceded by warm-up exercises and finished with a cool-down. Small, regular periods of exercise are far more efficient in toning the body than indulging in a long period of frantic movement once a week.

If you are deskbound at work, try to get up and walk about once every hour to stretch your limbs, and do a short series of stretching exercises daily. A daily, brisk, twenty-minute walk is a perfect first stage to fitness. There are many forms of exercise programmes available; the important thing is that you should choose the one that suits you best. Consider your physical abilities, age and the facilities available within your locality. Never rush into an exercise programme or go for the advanced exercises first. Start with gentle exercises and gradually work up to a routine that your body can cope with. If you have not taken part in any regular exercise for some time it is also a good idea to get the go-ahead from your regular doctor. No matter what your age, if your programme is a sensible one you will always improve with time.

HEALTHY MIND — HEALTHY BODY

Any mental stress will manifest itself within your body and show in your outward appearance. Many people, for example, acknowledge that they have a 'weak point' which is affected as soon as they experience stress. One person may develop a sore throat, another a headache, another an aching limb, all the result of some stressful occurrence. This is really nature's way of telling you that you have had enough and you should take time off. If you develop an ailment you have to stop and nurse yourself until you feel better. This is the resting time that your mind needs.

Stress is a natural function. The release of adrenaline into the bloodstream prepares us for 'fight or flight'. When we are in a dangerous situation or when suffering from shock, adrenaline helps us to cope. What is not productive is continual stress that takes a hold and will not go away.

The aim, then, is to reduce stress. When under stress you may feel alone and that no one can help you. Lesson number one is to care for yourself. Allow yourself the time to do something that makes you feel good. Go for a walk and look at the things around you.

Learning to relax
There are many relaxation techniques around and you can go to classes to learn them. Here is one that might help. Lie down on your back somewhere comfortable and warm, but not too hot. Close your eyes. Stretch all your limbs together and gradually let go. Do this twice. Imagine you are somewhere that you have enjoyed being, such as a beach or a grassy bank. Imagine the sun above you. Imagine its rays touching your body and warming you through. Think about

your feet. Flex them and relax them. Do the same with your lower legs, then the top of your legs, and gradually work your way up your body to the top of your head. Feel yourself to be weightless and imagine the golden glow of the sun penetrating your body. Apart from this, try to keep your mind blank. Lie there for as long as you can. When you want to finish, consciously feel each part of your body, from the toes up, keeping it relaxed but being aware of it.

Imagine the room that you are in and think of the floor or the earth beneath your feet. Slowly open your eyes.

MAKING YOUR OWN BEAUTY PREPARATIONS

Making your own beauty treatments is not difficult and you don't need a complicated range of equipment or ingredients. Many of the things you need can be found in the utensils and ingredients cupboards of the average, well-stocked kitchen, and the rest are easily bought.

What you cannot obtain are the chemical ingredients that are often to be found in even the most natural of shop-bought preparations. Nor do you have access to the whipping, stirring and mixing machinery that is used in most commercial manufacture. This means that the texture of your homemade creams may vary from bought ones, but this does not make them any less efficient or less of a joy to use. You can't expect them to be exactly the same, just as a homemade loaf of bread is rarely of a similar texture to a shop-bought one.

Before starting to make your own cosmetics, you must prepare a working area in your kitchen. As with cooking, you need some basic equipment, hot and cold running water, a power point and a stove. Give yourself plenty of room to work and clear the area of all food before you start mixing.

When making a recipe, have all the ingredients prepared (chopped, grated, etc.) and laid out on a table. Similarly, have all the necessary equipment ready before you begin.

EQUIPMENT

Opposite is a list of the equipment you will need to make the recipes in this book – you won't require every item for every single recipe. When starting to make your own cosmetics, use your usual kitchen equipment. If you decide that it is to become a hobby, consider keeping a separate set of basic equipment. This will avoid getting beeswax in the soup!

All your equipment should be clean before you begin, and your jars, containers and bottles sterilised. Even though they look clean, they may be harbouring a thin film of dust or dirt that could contaminate your new cosmetics or make them go mouldy.

To sterilise plastic containers, first make sure they are heat-resistant. Place them in a saucepan, cover with water and bring gently to the boil. Lift them out with tongs and let them drain. Dry with a clean cloth.

Glass containers can be sterilised in a low oven, about 40°C (100°F). Wash them first and place them on their side on the oven racks. Leave them for ten minutes. All lids and tops should be sterilised as well. Metal containers can be treated in the same way as plastic ones.

Important To prevent contamination from condensation, always allow the product you are making to cool completely before sealing it into its container.

USING HERBS

The most commonly used herbs are listed in the chart on page 19. Others are given in specific sections and recipes. Some dried herbs, such as chamomile and peppermint, can be bought from supermarkets in the form of herbal teas. More unusual ones, such as nettle or comfrey, must be bought from herbalists or healthfood shops. Herbs are most frequently made into infusions and decoctions, and recipes for these are given throughout the book.

CIDER VINEGAR

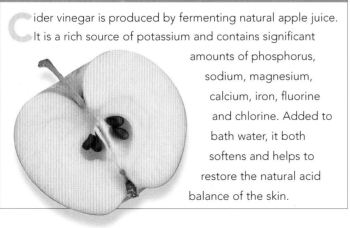

Cider vinegar is produced by fermenting natural apple juice. It is a rich source of potassium and contains significant amounts of phosphorus, sodium, magnesium, calcium, iron, fluorine and chlorine. Added to bath water, it both softens and helps to restore the natural acid balance of the skin.

INGREDIENTS

For the main ingredients that are used for skin care, refer to the chart on pages 20-21. Do not buy all the ingredients at once. Decide which recipes you would like to make and which ingredients are suitable for your skin type. Everybody's skin is different and reacts differently to certain ingredients and preparations. Before you go ahead and make a beauty treatment, do a 'patch test' to check whether you are allergic to any of the ingredients. The simplest way of doing this is to rub a little of the ingredient onto a part of your skin that is delicate but which does not show, such as the inside of your arm. Leave it for twelve hours.

If you have any sort of allergic reaction, do not use that particular ingredient. To check the effect of a herb, make up an infusion following the instructions on page 17 and dab it onto your skin in the same way.

A range of vegetable and nut oils is used in the book. Some, such as olive, coconut or sunflower, can be bought as foods. The rest can be bought from herbalists, healthfood shops, chemists and suppliers of essential oils for aromatherapy.

It is important to buy reputable brands of essential oils from aromatherapy suppliers or healthfood shops. In most cases, the more expensive the oils are, the better the quality, but it is worth getting advice from other users. There is more information on this topic on pages 98-99.

Other ingredients in the recipes that might be slightly less familiar include:

DECOCTION

Decoctions are usually greater in strength than infusions. The herb is put into a saucepan with cold water, brought to the boil and simmered for a given time. The liquid can be left to stand for a time after simmering or it can be immediately strained off. The amount of herb, the simmering time and the standing time can all affect strength. An average strength decoction is made by simmering 1 tbsp fresh chopped herb or 1 tsp dried in 300 ml (10 fl oz) water for ten minutes. It can then be strained immediately or left, covered, for ten minutes before straining.

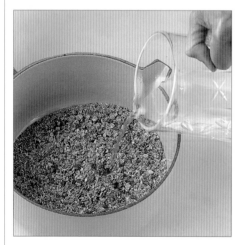

1 Fresh or dried herbs are placed in a stainless steel saucepan and covered with cold water.

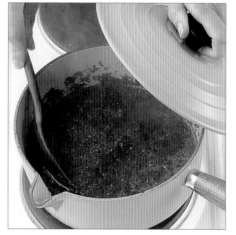

2 The mixture is brought to the boil, then simmered.

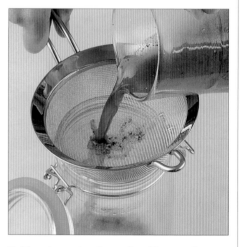

3 The decoction is strained into a clean container ready for use.

• *Arrowroot:* This is a white powder obtained by grinding the dried roots of the arrowroot plant. It is used to thicken sauces and other liquids, in a similar way to cornflour. It is used in teeth and hair preparations.

• *Beeswax:* This is the wax used by bees to make honey cells in the hive. Beeswax for cosmetic use has usually been purified by melting and straining. It is available in blocks, discs or sheets in its natural yellow colour or as discs in a purer white form. It can be obtained from honey producers, candle makers' suppliers and herbalists.

• *Borax:* Also known as sodium borate, borax is available as fine white crystals. It is added to washing water for its softening properties. Used very sparingly in beauty preparations, it will help to amalgamate the other ingredients.

• *Cocoa butter:* This is obtained by roasting and grinding cacao beans and then separating out the fat. Chocolate is what remains after the process. The pure 'butter' is sold in blocks. It is similar in texture to soap, but melts easily at a temperature of about 40°C (100°F).

INFUSION

Making an infusion is the same as making a cup of tea. An amount of the dried or fresh chopped herb is put into a container and boiling water is poured onto it. The mixture is covered, brewed for a while and then strained. Amounts and times are given in most recipes. The more herb that is used to a given amount of water and the longer it is left, the stronger the infusion. An average strength infusion is made with 1 tbsp fresh chopped herb or 1 tsp dried to 250 ml (8 fl oz) water.

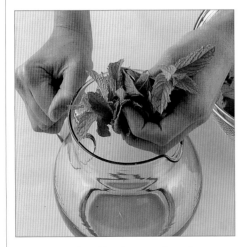

1 Fresh or dried herbs are placed in a heat-proof container.

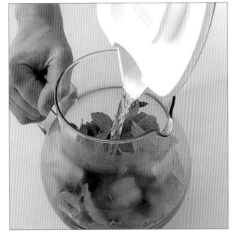

2 Boiling water is poured onto the herbs and the mixture covered and left to infuse.

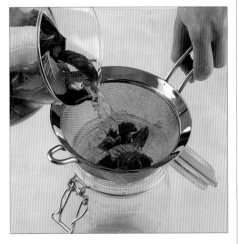

3 The cooled infusion is strained into a clean container ready for use.

Cocoa butter is available from herbalists and chemists.

• *Cultured buttermilk:* Buttermilk was originally the name given to the whey left in the churn after the butter had been made. Now it is the name for milk to which an acid culture has been added. Unlike yoghurt, it retains its liquid nature. If it is unavailable, use a thin, plain yoghurt for the recipes.

• *Fuller's earth:* This is a type of clay used in the textile industry for fulling (softening) cloth, that comes in the form of a fine, grey powder. It is available from herbalists and mail-order sources, and is perfectly harmless when used on the skin or hair. It acts as a carrier for other ingredients.

• *Glycerine:* This is a vegetable product, available as a clear, slightly thickened liquid. It is a natural moisturiser that helps to draw moisture from the lower skin area to the surface.

• *Kaolin powder:* This fine, white, powdered clay is used for making porcelain and can be found at ceramic supply shops. It has neutral properties and can be used as a carrier for other ingredients.

• *Lanolin:* This natural oil from sheep's wool is similar in composition to sebum, the natural oil on human skin. It has an emollient effect and also helps the skin to retain moisture. Lanolin is usually bought from chemists in the form of a rich, yellow-coloured, sticky cream.

• *Rosewater/orange flower water:* These fragrant waters are the by-products of the manufacture of the essential oils that come from rose and orange flowers. In the process, petals are subjected to concentrated steam which releases the essential oils. When the steam condenses, oil and water are separated. Rose and orange flower water are delicately scented and make natural skin fresheners.

• *Tincture of benzoin:* Benzoin is a resin that comes from the benzoin tree (*Styrax benzoin*). It is used in aromatic preparations, such as potpourris, as a fixative. A tincture is made by steeping it in alcohol. Used in beauty preparations, it has a tightening effect. Tincture of benzoin can be bought from good chemists and herbalists.

• *White petroleum jelly:* This is often marketed under the tradename Vaseline. It is a translucent, solid mixture of hydrocarbons, and is well-known for the soothing and softening effects it has on the skin.

• *Witch hazel:* Distilled witch hazel is a clear lotion produced from the twigs and bark of the witch hazel tree. It tones the skin, helping to close the pores. Witch hazel is a Native American healing herb that was adopted by early settlers and eventually taken to Europe.

Many different herbs are used in the recipes. If one is unavailable, you can often find an equally good substitute. This chart is intended as a guide to choosing the right herbs for your needs. As a general rule, oily skin needs astringent herbs that tighten and promote the closing of pores. Dry and mature skins need emollient herbs that will supplement the skin's own protective oils. All of these herbs soften, soothe and lubricate.

HERB	Anti-inflammatory	Antiseptic	Astringent	Cleansing	Emollient	Invigorating	Moisturizing	Soothing	Toning	SKIN TYPE Normal	Oily	Dry/Mature
Chamomile	✓			✓				✓	✓	✓	✓	✓
Comfrey					✓		✓	✓	✓	✓	✓	
Elderflower			✓	✓			✓	✓	✓	✓		✓
Fennel			✓	✓				✓	✓	✓	✓	
Lady's mantle					✓			✓	✓	✓		✓
Lavender		✓				✓		✓	✓	✓	✓	
Lemon balm								✓	✓	✓	✓	
Linden flowers				✓	✓		✓	✓	✓	✓		
Marigold			✓	✓			✓	✓	✓	✓	✓	✓
Marshmallow					✓			✓	✓	✓	✓	✓
Mint			✓					✓	✓		✓	
Nettle				✓		✓		✓	✓	✓	✓	✓
Parsley				✓				✓	✓	✓	✓	
Rosemary						✓		✓	✓	✓	✓	
Sage	✓		✓					✓	✓	✓	✓	
Thyme	✓			✓		✓		✓	✓	✓	✓	
Violet				✓	✓			✓	✓	✓	✓	
Witch hazel			✓					✓	✓	✓	✓	
Woodruff								✓	✓	✓	✓	
Yarrow			✓					✓	✓	✓	✓	

The food ingredients used for skin care preparations are easy to obtain. Most can be found in supermarkets and grocers. Others, such as brewer's yeast or bran, can be bought in healthfood shops. An ingredient under the heading **+ Acid** is one that helps to restore the acid balance of the skin. **Suncare** covers pre- and aftersun treatments.

	Cleansing	Exfoliant	Toning	Moisturizing	+ Acid	Softening	Suncare	Normal	Oily	Dry/Mature
Almond, ground	☐	☐	☐	☐		☐	☐	☐	☐	☐
Almond oil	☐			☐		☐	☐	☐		☐
Apricot			☐			☐	☐	☐	☐	☐
Apricot oil	☐			☐		☐	☐	☐		☐
Avocado	☐			☐		☐	☐	☐	☐	☐
Avocado oil	☐			☐		☐	☐	☐		☐
Banana						☐	☐	☐	☐	☐
Barley	☐	☐		☐		☐		☐	☐	☐
Beeswax	☐	☐		☐		☐		☐	☐	☐
Benzoin	☐							☐	☐	
Borax	☐					☐		☐	☐	☐
Bran		☐				☐		☐	☐	
Butter				☐		☐	☐	☐		☐
Buttermilk	☐	☐		☐	☐	☐	☐	☐	☐	
Cocoa butter	☐			☐		☐	☐	☐	☐	☐
Cornmeal	☐	☐	☐	☐		☐		☐	☐	☐
Cream, fresh				☐		☐	☐	☐		☐
Cream, sour				☐		☐	☐	☐		☐
Cucumber	☐		☐	☐	☐	☐	☐	☐	☐	☐
Egg white			☐			☐	☐	☐	☐	
Egg yolk				☐		☐	☐	☐		☐
Flower waters	☐							☐	☐	☐

	Cleansing	Exfoliant	Toning	Moisturising	+ Acid	Softening	Suncare	SKIN TYPE Normal	Oily	Dry/Mature
Fuller's earth								☐	☐	☐
Glycerine				☐				☐	☐	☐
Grape			☐	☐	☐	☐		☐	☐	☐
Grapefruit		☐	☐			☐		☐	☐	☐
Honey	☐		☐	☐		☐	☐	☐	☐	☐
Horseradish	☐		☐	☐	☐	☐		☐	☐	☐
Jojoba oil	☐			☐		☐	☐	☐	☐	☐
Lanolin	☐			☐		☐			☐	☐
Lemon	☐	☐	☐		☐	☐		☐	☐	☐
Milk				☐		☐	☐	☐		☐
Oatmeal	☐	☐	☐	☐		☐		☐	☐	
Olive oil	☐			☐		☐	☐			☐
Peach				☐		☐	☐	☐	☐	☐
Petroleum jelly	☐					☐		☐	☐	☐
Pineapple	☐	☐	☐		☐	☐		☐	☐	☐
Rice flour	☐	☐				☐		☐	☐	☐
Sea salt		☐						☐	☐	
Strawberry			☐	☐	☐	☐	☐	☐	☐	☐
Vinegar, cider	☐	☐	☐	☐	☐	☐		☐	☐	☐
Vinegar, wine	☐	☐	☐	☐	☐	☐		☐	☐	☐
Wheatgerm oil	☐			☐		☐	☐	☐		☐
Witch hazel	☐		☐			☐	☐	☐	☐	☐
Yoghurt	☐	☐	☐	☐	☐	☐	☐	☐	☐	☐

FACE

cleanse

exfoliate

tone

moisturise

nourish

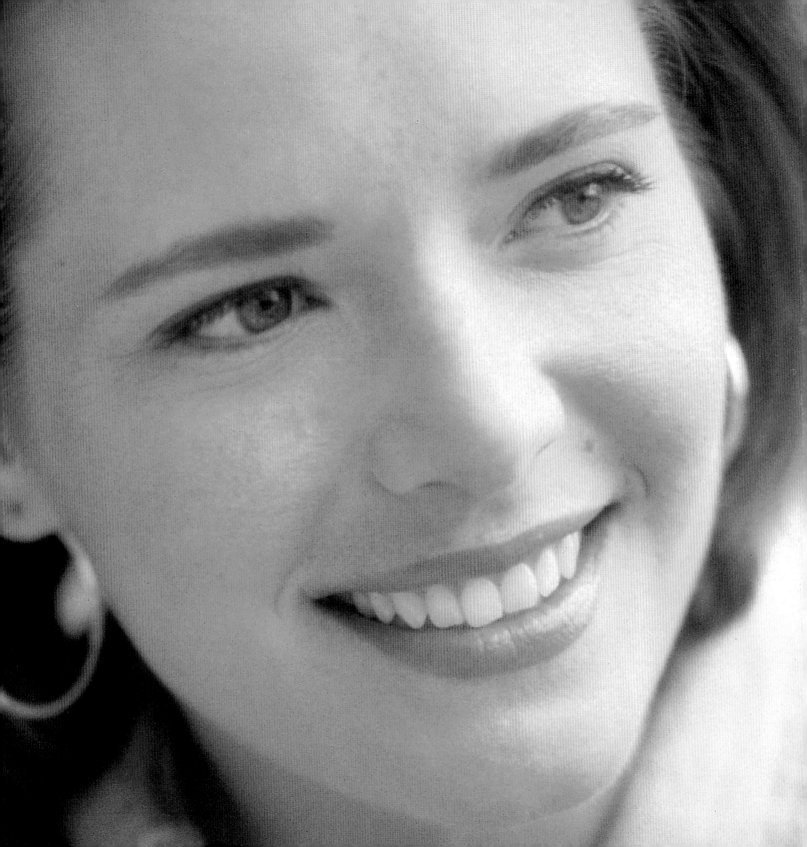

Your face is the part of you that you show to the world. It is also the part that is exposed to extremes of weather, to pollution, sunlight, and to the grime picked up through everyday living. You therefore have to make doubly sure that you take care of it.

The skin on a newborn baby is soft, smooth and very elastic, and there is a high turnover of cells. As we age, the parts of us most exposed to the outside world 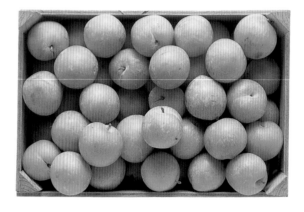 become coarser. This is largely due to the gradual slowing of the turnover of cells, which results in a build-up of dead cells on the surface of the skin. If we lavish plenty of time and attention on ourselves, some of the effects of ageing can be kept at bay.

Hormone changes throughout life can affect our skin. At adolescence, the effect is nearly always to produce excess sebum. It always seems unfair that just as you are starting to be attracted to the opposite sex, you are very often suffering from oily skin, blackheads or spots. During pregnancy skin seems to glow with health, but afterwards hormone changes again may cause it to be extra oily or extra dry. It is probably at menopause that women notice the greatest change to their skin, as its natural elasticity begins to weaken.

Never give up on your skin and your appearance. No matter how old you are, there is always something that you can do to improve your looks and to make yourself feel better.

FACIAL CARE

There are three basic, everyday steps to facial care. These are: cleansing, toning and moisturising. To this you can add: exfoliating, massage and exercise. All of these are explained in the pages that follow.

All the instructions and recipes in this book are for treatments, not for make-up. Whether you wear a heavy make-up every day consisting of foundation and powder, is up to you. If you do, extra emphasis must be put on cleansing. Wearing no make-up is good for your skin as it lets it breathe and keeps the pores free. Try to set aside certain days in the week when your skin can be as nature intended.

And don't forget your neck! It is just below your face and still on show, so look after it. Include it in your cleansing, toning and moisturising routine, and try the special treatments on page 47.

Remember that when you start a facial care treatment, the skin takes between three and four weeks to renew itself. You will probably have to wait that long to see clear results. Don't give up after a week or two because the treatment doesn't seem to be doing any good.

Assessing your skin type
Before you begin pampering your face, you must know what type of skin you have in order to choose the most suitable ingredients for your beauty preparations. Your basic skin type is usually inherited from your parents, but it is also affected by such things as diet, hormonal changes and the atmosphere of your surroundings. Whether your skin is dry, normal, oily or a combination type depends on how much sebum it produces.

Normal skin produces just enough sebum to keep the skin smooth and supple. Those people blessed with normal skin probably never even think about skin type, because their skin rarely poses a problem.

Oily skin produces more sebum than is needed; you may be able to feel a slight, greasy film on the surface. Where the sebaceous glands are over-productive, the acid mantle can become thick, clog the pores and produce blackheads or cause acne. Oily skin is particularly noticeable over what is called the T-zone, the part of the face comprising the central strip and the forehead. Monthly hormonal changes often affect oily skin. But oily skin can be kept under control, especially if it is exfoliated regularly and you pay particular attention to your diet. It also has the advantage of not ageing as quickly as dry or normal skin.

Dry skin is fine-textured and thin, and can become flaky and rough when exposed to extremes of temperature. It may be caused by insufficient sebum production or by dead cells on the surface failing to break up and so forming a scaly layer. That in turn encourages a loss of moisture from the cells coming up. Rich nourishing creams and gentle exfoliation help.

Combination skin is a combination of normal and oily skin, the oily area being in the above mentioned T-zone. Each of the recipes is coded so that you can tell at a glance which ones will suit your skin: **N** normal, **D** dry, **O** oily, **P** problem and **A** all types.

CLEANSING

By the end of a busy day, the skin on your face will have picked up a good deal of grime from the atmosphere, which mixes with dead skin cells, sebum, sweat and any make-up you are wearing. If you did not cleanse your skin, every day more matter would build up, your pores would become clogged, and your skin would become dull and lifeless. Even traces of dirt left behind can cause problems, so proper daily cleansing should be built into your routine.

A quick splash with warm water will not be sufficient, although it is a good start and helps to get off the surface grime. Many people swear by soap and water, but soaps are often very alkaline and destroy the acid mantle of the skin. If you like soap, choose one that is gentle and specially made for the face.

Cleansing creams and oils are excellent for removing make-up and most of the daily grime, and are mostly suitable for normal and dry skins. They do, however, leave a thin film of oil behind, so you should also use a facial scrub or steam from time to time. Oily skins need something lighter and oil-free.

Steaming

Along with everyday cleansing, your face needs a more thorough cleansing at regular intervals. Steaming is an excellent way of softening the skin and opening the pores to rid them of excess sebum. It can also soften blackheads, making them easier to remove. Even dry skin can benefit from steaming, particularly if it is followed by a massage using a nourishing oil.

The steam from plain water can moisturise and soften your skin. However, if the boiling water is poured over dried or chopped herbs, the properties of the herbs will be released.

It is best not to steam too frequently since, after all, it does subject your delicate facial skin to an unusual heat. Once a week is fine for normal or oily skin; every two weeks if you have dry skin. Do not steam your face if you have broken veins. See page 33 for instructions on how best to steam and deep clean your skin.

HERBS FOR STEAMING

Choose one of the following herbs or refer to the chart on page 19.

All skin types
Chamomile, comfrey, elderflower, linden flower, nettle

Normal or dry skin
Lady's mantle, marshmallow

Normal or oily skin
Fennel, lemon balm, rosemary

Oily skin
Sage, mint, yarrow

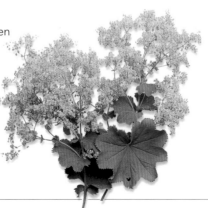

Gently massage one of these simple skin cleansers into the skin, then rinse off with lukewarm water or a herbal infusion chosen to suit your skin type.

• Buttermilk; cornmeal, ground almonds or fine oatmeal made into a paste with mineral water; plain yoghurt on its own or mixed with a little herbal infusion (all skin types); for oily skin, mix plain yoghurt with a little lemon juice; use dried milk powder, moistened with water on normal or oily skin, and whole milk on normal or dry skin.

RECIPE

HERBAL WITCH HAZEL CLEANSER Ⓐ

A light, liquid cleansing lotion that is excellent for wiping away daily grime. Soak a cotton wool ball in the lotion and wipe it gently over your face. Choose a herb to suit your skin type.

1 tsp dried or 1 tbsp fresh chopped chosen herb

100 ml (3 fl oz) boiling water

4 tbsp witch hazel

2 tbsp glycerine

1 Place the herb in a bowl and pour on the boiling water. Cover and leave to cool. Strain.
2 Pour 2 tbsp of the infusion into a sterilised bottle or jar. Add the witch hazel and glycerine. Cover tightly and shake well.
3 Store in a refrigerator and use within one week. Shake before use.

RECIPE

BUTTERMILK AND HONEY CLEANSER Ⓝ Ⓓ

Buttermilk is very soothing for the face. The herbs used here are for normal to dry skin. For an oily skin, use yarrow, sage or horsetail, or a mixture of two of them.

150 ml (5 fl oz) buttermilk

1 tsp dried or 1 tbsp fresh elderflowers

1 tsp dried or 1 tbsp fresh linden flowers

1 tsp honey

1 Place the buttermilk and herbs in a saucepan. Cover and leave for two hours.
2 Set the pan on a low heat and bring the mixture gently to the boil.
3 Remove from the heat, stir in the honey and leave to cool.
4 Strain off the liquid and pour it into a sterilised bottle. Seal and store in a refrigerator. Use within five days.

LINDEN OR LIME TREE (*Tilea vulgaris*)

Linden or lime trees grow wild and in parks and gardens throughout the northern temperate zones of the world. Infusions and decoctions of linden flowers are very emollient and can be used for all skin types.

Linden trees are common in Britain and Europe. Three species of linden (*Tilea*) are cultivated in Australia and New Zealand, while two species of lime (*Citrus*) are also available.

Other traditional names for the linden are lime tree, line, linn flowers, pry and whitewood.

The sweetly scented yellow-green flowers of the linden are usually ready for picking and drying in midsummer. You can sometimes buy dried linden flowers, but if they are unavailable, buy linden flower tea bags. (Make sure that no other ingredients have been added to the tea bags.)

MILK AND CUCUMBER CLEANSER Ⓝ ◎

This cleanser is for normal to oily skin. It is cooling and refreshing and leaves your skin feeling very smooth.

5 cm (2 in) piece cucumber

100 ml (3 fl oz) milk

4 drops tincture of benzoin

1 Peel and chop the cucumber.
2 Place the cucumber in a blender or food processor. Add the milk and work until smooth.
3 Pour the mixture into a saucepan and set on a medium heat. Bring to simmering point and hold there for two minutes.
4 Remove from the heat and allow to cool. Strain.
5 Pour the liquid into a sterilised bottle and add the tincture of benzoin.
6 Store in a refrigerator and use within one week.

YOGHURT CLEANSER Ⓐ

Yoghurt acts as a skin food as well as a cleanser, and leaves your skin feeling smooth. Choose a herb to suit your skin type.

1 tsp dried or 1 tbsp fresh chopped chosen herb

100 ml (3 fl oz) boiling water

5 tbsp plain yoghurt

1 tsp lemon juice (for oily skin)

1 tsp wheatgerm oil (for dry to normal skin)

1 Place the herb in a bowl and pour on the boiling water. Cover and leave to cool. Strain.
2 Place the yoghurt in a bowl and gradually beat in the infusion. Add the lemon juice or wheatgerm oil.
3 Store in a sterilised jar in a refrigerator and use within one week. Shake before using, especially if using oil.

ALMOND MILK CLEANSER Ⓐ

Almond milk is a time-honoured beauty treatment. Crushing the almonds by hand is said to draw out more 'milk', but you can use a blender or food processor instead. The cleanser is suitable for all skin types.

6 tbsp whole almonds

cold water

2 tsp honey

200 ml (6 ½ fl oz) mineral water

4 tbsp rosewater

1 Place the almonds in a saucepan and cover them with cold water. Bring to the boil. Allow to cool. Strain, then squeeze the almonds from their skins when still moist.
2 Chop the almonds finely by hand or in a blender or food processor.
3 Crush the almonds by hand using a large, heavy mortar and pestle.
4 Transfer the almonds to a bowl and beat in the honey. Add the mineral water, a few tablespoons at a time. Cover and leave to stand for eight hours.
5 Strain off the liquid through muslin, squeezing well to extract as much as possible.
6 Add the rosewater.
7 Store in a sterilised bottle or jar in a refrigerator. Use within three weeks.

ALMONDS

In medieval times, almond milk, made by soaking, simmering and straining pulverised almonds, was used for both culinary and beauty purposes when ordinary milk was scarce. This was often the case during the winter months or during Lent, when the use of cow's milk was forbidden.

SOAPWORT CLEANSER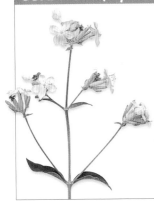

Keep in the bathroom and use directly from the bottle, as a gentle facewash. It will lather like soap but will leave your skin feeling soft. After use, rinse with warm water and pat dry.

1 tbsp soapwort root

2 tbsp dried or 6 tbsp fresh chopped chosen herb

1.5 litres (2 ½ pints) water, preferably mineral water

1 Place the soapwort root and herb in a saucepan with the water and cover. Bring gently to the boil and simmer for five minutes.
2 Take the pan from the heat and leave the decoction to cool.
3 Strain, pressing down well, and bottle the liquid. Use within one month.

SOAPWORT (Saponaria officinalis) AND SOAPBARK (Quillaja saponaria)

Soapwort is the mildest form of cleanser for any skin type. When the dried root is simmered in water, it produces a decoction that will lather slightly when used as a wash. It can safely be used as a substitute for face and body soap or as a wash for the hair.

Soapbark can be used in the same ways as soapwort. The bark of the tree produces a foamy liquid when boiled. It was once used to make foamy soft drinks, but is now just used externally and as a fabric cleaner. Soapbark grows in South America, most particularly in Chile, and is a member of the wing-seeded section of the rose family. It is an evergreen tree with thick, toothed, oval, shiny green leaves and white flowers. It can grow up to 18 metres (60 feet) high and is also known as Panama Bark Tree and Cullay.

COCOA BUTTER CLEANSER

This is an excellent lotion for dry skin. It enriches and moisturises the area around the eyes as it cleanses. Mineral water may be used instead of the elderflower infusion.

1 tbsp elderflowers

150 ml (5 fl oz) boiling water

1 tbsp cocoa butter

1 tbsp lanolin

125 ml (4 fl oz) almond or olive oil

1 Place the elderflowers in a jug and pour on the boiling water. Cover and leave to cool. Strain.
2 Place the cocoa butter, lanolin and oil in the top of a double boiler or in a bowl set in a saucepan of water. Melt together over a low heat.
3 Remove the mixture from the heat and add 3 tbsp of the elderflower infusion.
4 Whisk the mixture until it is well blended and cool.
5 Transfer the lotion to a sterilised pot or jar. Cover when completely cold. Use within three months.

LIGHT BEESWAX CLEANSER

This is a light-textured cleansing cream, suitable for all skin types. For normal and dry skin use rosewater or an infusion of elderflowers or marigolds; for oily skin, use chamomile or yarrow.

1 tbsp beeswax

1 tbsp white petroleum jelly

4 tbsp almond oil

2 tbsp rosewater or herbal infusion

2-3 drops essential oil such as rose or lavender (only if using infusion)

1 Place the beeswax, petroleum jelly and almond oil in the top of a double boiler or in a bowl set in a saucepan of water. Melt them gently together on a low heat.
2 Warm the rosewater or infusion.
3 Remove entirely from the heat and beat the rosewater or infusion into the beeswax mixture. Leave to cool.
4 Transfer the cream to a sterilised pot or jar. Cover when completely cold. Use within three months.

ALMOND AND IRISH MOSS CLEANSER ⊙

In texture this is rather like soft modelling clay, and spreads easily over the face. Spread it on with your fingers and remove with soft tissues or cotton wool balls.

150 ml (5 fl oz) hot water

½ tsp borax

2 tsp Irish moss

1 tbsp almond oil

2 tbsp ground almonds

1 In a bowl, dissolve the borax in the hot water.
2 Add the Irish moss and leave to soak for four hours or until it becomes soft and jelly-like.
3 Mix together the almonds and oil.
4 Stir them vigorously into the Irish moss.
5 Store in a sterilised pot or jar in a refrigerator. Use within two weeks.

IRISH MOSS (*Chondrus crispus*)

Irish moss, or carragheen, is a seaweed that grows in purple-brown fan shapes on rocks or in rock pools below the tide line. It is harvested in the spring and dried. When mixed with water and soaked or simmered, it forms a jelly-like mucilage that can be used as a base for desserts or for medicinal and beauty purposes.

HERBAL COLD CREAM Ⓐ

The ancient recipe for cold cream has remained the same for nearly 2,000 years. It is suitable for all skin types, particularly if a herbal infusion to match your skin is used as the liquid.

1 tbsp dried chosen herb to suit skin

150 ml (5 fl oz) boiling water

¼ tsp borax

1 tbsp beeswax

100 ml (3 fl oz) almond oil

1 drop rose or other suitable essential oil

1 Place the herb in a jug and pour in the boiling water. Cover and leave to cool slightly. Strain.
2 Dissolve the borax in 4 tbsp of the warm infusion.
3 Place the wax and oil in the top of a double boiler or in a bowl set in a saucepan of water. Set on a low heat and melt the wax and oil.
4 Beat in the infusion, then add the rose or other essential oil.
5 Remove entirely from the heat and beat vigorously with a wooden spoon or an electric beater, until the mixture is cool and creamy in texture.
6 Transfer the cream to a sterilised pot or jar. Cover when completely cold. Use within three months.

COLD CREAM

Cold cream was invented by Galen, personal physician to the Emperor Marcus Aurelius around AD 170. In the sixteenth century it was prepared with oil of cole-seed and called 'cole cream', which later became 'cold cream'. It has been used as a moisturiser and a cleanser and, in the sixteenth century, it was spread on cloth and used as a night-time face mask.

APRICOT AND AVOCADO CLEANSER Ⓝ Ⓓ

This light-textured cream should be used at night as a combined cleanser and enriching oil. Leave the residue to nourish your skin as you sleep.

4 tbsp apricot oil

4 tbsp avocado oil

2 tbsp chosen herbal infusion or mineral water

1 Beat all the ingredients together with an electric beater. The mixture should be light, white and creamy in texture.
2 Transfer to a sterilised bottle or jar and cover. Shake well before use. Use within two months.

RICH MARIGOLD CLEANSER Ⓝ Ⓓ

This makes a very soft cream that is suitable for normal or dry, sensitive skins.

4 fresh or dried marigold heads

1 tbsp cocoa butter

1 tbsp lanolin

125 ml (4 fl oz) almond, avocado, apricot or olive oil

1 Place all the ingredients in the top of a double boiler or in a bowl set in a pan of water. Set them on a low heat and let the cocoa butter, lanolin and oil melt together.
2 Leave on a low heat for a further five minutes.
3 Strain the mixture through a sieve into another bowl and beat until it cools.
4 Transfer the cream to a sterilised pot or jar. Cover when completely cold. Use within three months.

MARIGOLD (*Calendula officinalis*)

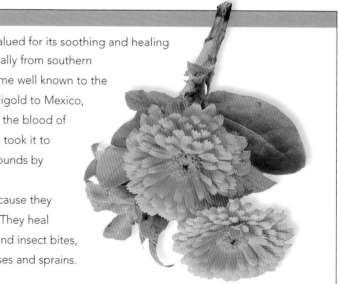

The marigold, or calendula, has been valued for its soothing and healing properties for centuries. It came originally from southern Europe, but was soon taken north to become well known to the Anglo-Saxons. The Spaniards took the marigold to Mexico, where it was believed to have sprung from the blood of natives killed by the invaders. Early settlers took it to North America; it was later used to heal wounds by both sides in the American Civil War.

Marigolds have always been popular because they are easy to grow and exceptionally useful. They heal wounds, soothe chilblains (see page 114) and insect bites, and can be made into a compress for bruises and sprains.

EXFOLIATING

Exfoliation is the process by which unwanted dead cells are removed from the surface of the skin to encourage new growth and a healthy glow. The value of exfoliants for all skin types has been recognised only in the last few years.

Five hundred million dead cells rub off us daily, and it has been found that gently assisting their departure helps to speed up the production of new cells and improve blood circulation in the skin. So if your skin looks dull and uneven, remove the top layer with a mild exfoliant to make it smooth, shiny and glowing.

Unless you have a medical skin complaint, you will benefit from exfoliation. A dry skin, for example, is often only dry because the outer layer of dead cells cling persistently together and cannot break down. If you give it a regular helping hand, the skin's surface will no longer be dry and may become normal.

It is never too late to begin exfoliating your skin. If you get into the habit early, then your skin will benefit for the rest of your life. As you get older, the rate of cell replacement in your skin slows down naturally, but regular exfoliation will give it a boost and may keep you looking younger for a little longer.

If you have never tried an exfoliant on your skin before, it is best to start with the milder ingredients such as oatmeal, buttermilk and ground almonds. If your skin benefits from the treatment and there are no ill effects, try adding small amounts of fruit, such as pineapple or lemon, to find the ingredients that suit you best.

Face masks

Homemade face masks have many uses, both direct and indirect. They have a beneficial effect on the skin of the face which can be cleansing, moisturising, healing, tightening or exfoliating. Their secondary effect is brought about by the fact that you generally have to lie down while they take effect. If you walk about, they may slither downwards. You can't even talk when wearing those that harden on the skin. So relax, lie down and make this a part of the treatment, too.

Face masks have to be of a spreadable consistency that will stay on the face. Some, as mentioned above, are designed to dry and harden, others change very little. They are all made from a base substance into which other ingredients are mixed.

Base substances include cereals, such as oatmeal, cornmeal, rice flour, barley and bran, and natural powders, such as fuller's earth or

EXFOLIATION

What you will need:

Bowl large enough to hold 600 ml (1 pint) boiling water

1 tbsp dried or 3 tbsp fresh chopped herbs

Face mask or scrub chosen from the recipes found on pages 35-36

2-3 medium-sized towels

Face cloth

Toner and moisturiser chosen to suit skin type

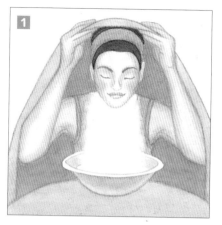

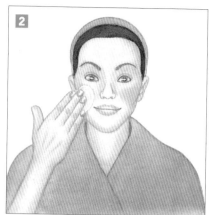

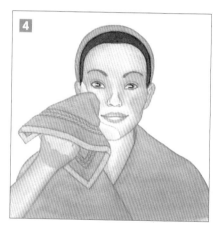

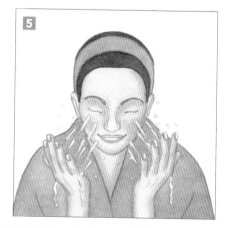

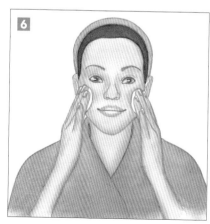

1 Place the herb in the bowl and pour on the boiling water. Cover your head and the bowl with the towel and close your eyes. Keep your face 30 cm (1 ft) above the water for 10-15 minutes.

2 Prepare your chosen scrub or mask, then tie back your hair and wrap a towel around your shoulders. Using the tips of your fingers, spread the mixture in an even layer over your face and neck, avoiding the sensitive part around your eyes. If you have chosen a scrub, massage it into your skin then go to step 4.

3 If using a face mask, lie down and relax for 15 minutes. (First cover a pillow with another towel.) Breathe deeply and enjoy this special time.

4 Wipe away the scrub. When the mask treatment is finished, come back to the world slowly. Gently wipe away the mask with a face cloth.

5 Rinse off the remaining mask or scrub with lukewarm water and pat your face dry.

6 Apply a toner and then a suitable moisturiser while your skin is still slightly damp.

kaolin. Ground almonds could also be included in this section. These are dry and powdery and have to be moistened. Moisteners include small amounts of natural oils, dairy products such as buttermilk, milk, yoghurt or cream, egg (either whole or separated), fruit or vegetable purées or herbal infusions.

Exfoliants can be used either as a facial scrub or as a mask. A scrub is useful when time is short, a mask takes longer and is more relaxing. For a deep-cleansing effect, steam your face first.

TONING

After cleansing, steaming or exfoliating, the skin must be toned to cool it down and help it to contract. Toners reduce any grease left behind by oil-based cleansers; they help to dry oily skin and leave it feeling cool and fresh.

MOISTURISING

Water is essential in maintaining a healthy skin. Drinking eight glasses of water a day will help, but you can also add moisture from the outside. A good moisturising treatment should both moisturise and nourish. It should add water to the skin's surface and should also help to reinforce the thin oily layer on the skin called the hydrolipidic film, which helps to keep the moisture from disappearing into the surrounding atmosphere.

Moisturising comes after cleansing and toning. It is a good idea to massage the moisturiser into your skin before the toner is completely dry, thus keeping in even more moisture. Spread the mixture onto your face with your fingertips, using some of the facial

(Continued on page 38.)

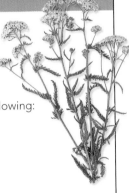

HERBS FOR TONING

Normal skin

Chamomile, dandelion, elderflower, fennel, lemon balm, marigold, parsley, rosemary

Oily skin

Choose from herbs listed for normal skin or any of the following: horsetail, lady's mantle, peppermint, sage, yarrow

Dry skin

Elderflower, linden flowers, marigold, marshmallow (mix the infusion half and half with rosewater.)

OATMEAL

Oatmeal has been used for centuries as a natural cleanser and softener. When moistened and rubbed into the skin it dislodges surface cells and embedded dirt as well as cleansing the pores. It also contains proteins that nourish and soften the skin at the same time. Oatmeal is a very mild skin treatment that can be used on all skin types, including sensitive skins and on skins that have acne.

RECIPE — GROUND ALMOND AND HONEY FACIAL SCRUB Ⓐ

This is a mild exfoliant and a good one to start with. The rose oil is not essential, but it makes a luxurious preparation if added. Do not use a synthetic rose oil.

2 tbsp ground almonds

2 tsp honey

4 tbsp buttermilk or plain yoghurt

2 drops rose oil

1 Place the ground almonds and honey in a bowl.
2 Mix in the buttermilk to make a thick paste.
3 Beat in the rose oil.
4 Gently massage the mixture into your face and neck for about two minutes, avoiding the area directly around the eyes.
5 Rinse off the mixture with tepid water. Pat dry, tone and moisturise.

RECIPE — HERBAL FACIAL SCRUB Ⓐ

This is very mild and gentle, and so another good scrub to begin with.

herbal infusion made with chamomile, elderflowers or fennel

2 tbsp fine oatmeal

1 Mix 3 tbsp of the infusion with the oatmeal to make a paste. Leave the oatmeal to soften for five minutes.
2 Gently massage the mixture into your face for five minutes.
3 Rinse off the mixture with tepid water. Pat dry, tone and moisturise.

RECIPE — OATMEAL AND YOGHURT FACIAL SCRUB Ⓓ Ⓟ

The almond oil makes this an ideal scrub for dry skin, leaving it feeling soft and smooth. Without the almond oil, the exfoliant is suitable for skin that suffers from acne.

2 tbsp fine oatmeal

2 tbsp plain yoghurt

1 tbsp almond oil

1 Place the oatmeal in a bowl and gradually mix in the yoghurt and almond oil. Leave the oatmeal to soften for five minutes.
2 Gently massage the mixture into your face and neck for about five minutes, avoiding the area directly around the eyes.
3 Rinse off with tepid water, pat dry, tone and moisturise.

RECIPE — CORNMEAL FACIAL SCRUB ◎

Cornmeal exfoliators are good for oily skins, and the lemon juice adds to the acid mantle.

2 tbsp cornmeal

1 tsp lemon juice

2 tbsp plain yoghurt or buttermilk

1 Place the cornmeal in a bowl.
2 Mix in the lemon juice and buttermilk to make a paste. Leave the cornmeal to soften for five minutes.
3 Gently massage the paste into your face for about five minutes, avoiding the area around the eyes.
4 Rinse off the mixture with tepid water. Pat dry, tone and moisturise.

RECIPE — GRAPEFRUIT AND PARSLEY FACE MASK ◎

This leaves your skin feeling new and refreshed. Parsley is particularly good for oily skin.

3 tbsp fine oatmeal

2 tbsp chopped parsley

juice of ½ large grapefruit

1 Place the oatmeal and parsley in a bowl.
2 Mix in enough grapefruit juice to make a spreadable paste. Let soften for five minutes.
3 Spread the mixture evenly over your face.
4 Lie down and relax for 15 minutes.
5 Rinse off the mixture with tepid water. Pat dry, tone and moisturise.

PINEAPPLE AND CORNMEAL FACE MASK ◎

Pineapple leaves your skin feeling fresh and slightly tight. Like the previous cornmeal recipe, this is good for oily skin.

1 slice pineapple, 13 mm (½ in) thick

2 tbsp plain yoghurt

4 tbsp cornmeal

1 Purée the pineapple slice in a food processor or blender.
2 Put the purée in a bowl and mix in the yoghurt and enough cornmeal to make a thick paste. Leave it for five minutes for the cornmeal to soften.
3 Spread the paste over your face, avoiding the area immediately around the eyes.
4 Lie down and relax for 15 minutes.
5 Rinse off the mixture with tepid water, pat dry, tone and moisturise.

PINEAPPLE

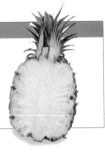

Pineapple is a natural exfoliant. It contains a protein-digesting enzyme called bromelin that gently breaks down the dead skin cells so they can be easily removed, leaving your skin feeling soft and smooth. Pineapple also restores the skin's natural acid mantle. Pineapple slices can be puréed and made into face masks or scrubs. You can also lay thin slices on your face while you lie down and relax.

HERBAL MILK TONER ◎ ℗

Skin toners made with milk are soothing and nourishing for dry, sunburned or sensitive skins. Choose whole milk for dry or normal skin, skimmed milk for oily skin.

2 tsp dried or 1 tbsp fresh chopped herb chosen to suit skin type

150 ml (5 fl oz) milk

1 Place the herb in a bowl or jug.
2 Boil the milk and pour it over the herb. Cover and leave until cold.
3 Strain through muslin or cheesecloth.
4 Store in a sterilised bottle or jar in a refrigerator. Use within five days.

HERB AND WITCH HAZEL TONER ◎

This is a light, refreshing toner for all skin types that is very easy to make.

1 tsp dried or 1 tbsp fresh chopped herb chosen to suit skin type

100 ml (3 fl oz) boiling water

2 tbsp witch hazel

pinch boric acid

1 Place the herb in a bowl or jug and pour on the boiling water. Cover and leave to cool. Strain.
2 Mix the boric acid into the witch hazel.
3 Add the witch hazel to the herbal infusion.
4 Store in a sterilised bottle or jar in a refrigerator and use within one month. Shake well before use.

EGG WHITE AND LEMON TONER ◎

This is a toner for oily skin.

1 tbsp dried or 2 tbsp fresh chopped yarrow, horsetail or sage

150 ml (5 fl oz) boiling water

1 egg white

juice ½ lemon, strained

1 Place the herb in a jug or bowl and pour on the boiling water. Cover and leave to cool. Strain.
2 Whisk the egg white and lemon juice together.
3 Mix in the herbal infusion.
4 Store in a sterilised bottle or jar in a refrigerator. Use within one week.

• The simplest toner is cold water, rosewater or orange flower water, or a cold herbal infusion. Other things to wipe on your face include a slice of cucumber or the inside of a cucumber peel (all skin types); a cut strawberry (normal or oily skin). You may need to wash off any strawberry stains left on your skin, but the other toners can be left to dry.

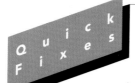

RECIPE

CITRUS TONER ⓝ ◎

This is a deliciously scented toner that freshens and clears normal to oily skin.

peel from 2 lemons, 2 oranges and 1 grapefruit

300 ml (10 fl oz) mineral water

2 tbsp vodka (optional, but it doubles the shelflife)

1 Place the citrus peels in a jug or bowl and pour on the mineral water. Cover and leave for 12 hours.
2 Strain the liquid through a coffee filter and into a sterilised bottle or jar. Add the vodka. Store in a refrigerator and use within two weeks (four weeks if vodka is added).

RECIPE

ALMOND TONER ◎

This is an astringent toner, good for oily skin.

150 ml (5 fl oz) rosewater

½ tsp borax

1 tsp tincture of benzoin

1 tsp ground almonds

3 tbsp mineral water or distilled water

1 Place the rosewater in a sterilised bottle or jar.
2 Dissolve the borax in the tincture of benzoin and add to the rosewater.
3 Mix the almonds with the water and add to the rosewater. Shake well.
4 Store in a refrigerator and use within one month. Shake before using.

RECIPE

CUCUMBER AND ELDERFLOWER TONER ⓐ

This cooling and refreshing toner can be used for all skin types. The vodka prevents the cucumber from going mouldy.

1 cucumber

3 tbsp dried elderflowers or 3 fresh heads

125 ml (4 fl oz) boiling water

100 ml (3 fl oz) vodka

1 Slice the cucumber. Place the slices in a saucepan with no water and set them on a low heat. Simmer until soft. Allow to cool, then strain off the liquid through muslin, squeezing to extract as much liquid as possible.
2 Place the elderflowers in a jug or bowl and pour on the boiling water. Cover and leave to cool. Strain off the infusion.
3 Add the vodka and the infusion to the cucumber juice. Store in a refrigerator and use within two weeks.

CUCUMBER

The cucumber contains a large proportion of water, and so is naturally moisturising. It also has the same acid–alkaline balance as the skin itself, making it one of the gentlest and most balanced of beauty treatments. Cucumber is used to moisturise and tone, and to ease sunburn and the effects of the weather.

massage techniques shown on page 50. Remember to moisturise your neck as well.

If you have normal skin, use a light moisturiser in the daytime and a richer one for overnight.

If you live and work in air-conditioned areas, or if you spend a lot of your time outdoors, you are more likely to have dry skin. Dry skins often do not produce enough sebum to maintain the acid mantle, so twice daily nourishing and moisturising are particularly important. Use rich, oil-based moisturisers, and consider patting extra wheatgerm or another natural vegetable oil into the skin at night after using the moisturiser.

Oily skin may not need moisturising twice a day or even every day. As a replacement use a toner that moisturises but which is not too astringent, and let it dry naturally. Examples are those made from one of the emollient herbs, such as linden flower or elderflower, or from rosewater and witch hazel. Try 'Herb and witch hazel', 'Cucumber and elderflower' or 'Almond' from the toner recipes on pages 36-37.

When you need to moisturise, use a light moisturising lotion. If you have been out in the sun and wind all day and your skin feels dry, do use a rich moisturiser or massage in some jojoba or avocado oil.

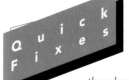

Quick Fixes

If the skin on your face feels slack, try a face mask that will both tone and tighten.
- For very oily skin, beat the egg white with either 1 tbsp lemon juice or cider vinegar.
- For normal or dry skin, apply a lightly beaten egg white and leave it to dry on your face. Adding 1 tbsp skimmed milk powder will soften your skin; 1 tsp honey will moisturise.
- Add 2 tbsp fresh chopped herbs to the beaten white; for example, parsley for normal skin and mint for oily skin.

RECIPE **CUCUMBER AND COCONUT MOISTURISER** Ⓝ Ⓓ

This soft, pale-green cream is suitable for dry or normal skins. You can feel the moisture of the cucumber as you spread it over your face.

7.5 cm (3 in) piece cucumber

pinch borax

1 tsp lanolin

1 tsp cocoa butter

1 tbsp beeswax

2 tbsp coconut oil

1 Finely chop the cucumber and press it in a sieve to extract the juice. There should be about 2 tbsp.
2 Warm the juice and dissolve the borax in it.
3 Place the lanolin, cocoa butter, beeswax and coconut oil in the top of a double boiler or in a bowl set in a saucepan of water. Melt on a low heat.
4 Remove entirely from the heat and beat in the cucumber juice until the mixture is cool.
5 Transfer the cream to a sterilised pot or jar. Cover when completely cold. Use within six weeks.

VITAMIN-ENRICHED MOISTURISER Ⓝ Ⓓ

Use this rich, creamy-textured, yellow moisture cream for dry or normal skin types under make-up or overnight. Rosewater can be substituted for the herbal decoction.

1 tsp dried or 1 tbsp fresh chopped herb chosen to suit skin type

150 ml (5 fl oz) water

2 tbsp lanolin

2 tbsp beeswax

2 tbsp wheatgerm oil

100 ml (3 fl oz) almond, avocado or olive oil

one 250 iu capsule vitamin E

one 250 iu capsule vitamin A

3 drops essential oil such as rose, lavender or geranium (optional)

1 Place the herb and water in a saucepan and bring to the boil. Cover and simmer for five minutes. Leave to cool, then strain off the decoction.
2 Place the lanolin and beeswax in the top of a double boiler or in a bowl set in a saucepan of water. Melt gently on a low heat.
3 Gradually beat in the oils.
4 Remove entirely from the heat and beat in 2 tbsp of the herbal decoction or rosewater.
5 Pierce the vitamin capsules and squeeze the contents into the cream. Beat well, adding the essential oil, if using.
6 Cool, stirring frequently.
7 Transfer the cream to a sterilised pot or jar. Cover when completely cold. Use within two months.

COCOA BUTTER MOISTURISER Ⓓ

Rosewater can be substituted for the herbal decoction in this rich, fairly stiff cream.

1 tsp dried or 1 tbsp fresh chopped herb chosen to suit skin type

150 ml (5 fl oz) water

3 tbsp cocoa butter

1 tbsp beeswax

125 ml (4 fl oz) almond, avocado, olive or safflower oil

3 drops essential oil such as rose, lavender or geranium (optional)

1 Place the herb and water in a saucepan and bring to the boil. Cover and simmer for five minutes. Leave to cool, then strain off the decoction.
2 Place the cocoa butter and beeswax in the top of a double boiler or in a bowl set in a saucepan of water. Melt gently on a low heat.
3 Gradually beat in the oil.
4 Remove entirely from the heat and beat in 2 tbsp of the herbal decoction or rosewater. Add the essential oil, if using.
5 Cool, stirring frequently.
6 Transfer the cream to a sterilised pot or jar. Cover when completely cold. Use within two months.

GERANIUM OIL

Geranium oil is revitalising and relaxing. It is produced, mainly in countries around the Mediterranean, by a steam distillation of the leaves and flowers of a species of pelargonium.

The scent of geranium oil combines a herbal freshness with an underlying sweetness, and it is often used to scent soaps, creams and perfumes.

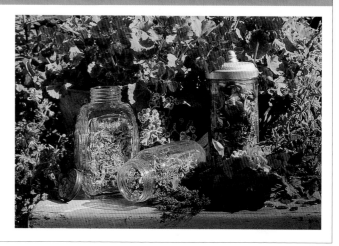

HONEY AND OLIVE OIL MOISTURISER Ⓝ Ⓓ

This light-coloured cream suits dry or normal skin. Rosewater can be substituted for the herbal infusion.

1 tsp dried or 1 tbsp fresh chopped herb chosen to suit skin type

150 ml (5 fl oz) water

1 tbsp beeswax

2 tbsp lanolin

100 ml (3 fl oz) olive oil

2 tsp honey

2 drops essential oil such as rose, lavender or geranium (optional)

1 Place the herb and water in a saucepan and bring to the boil. Cover and simmer for five minutes. Leave to cool, then strain off the decoction.
2 Place the beeswax and lanolin in the top of a double boiler or in a bowl set in a saucepan of water. Melt gently on a low heat.
3 Gradually beat in the oil.
4 Remove entirely from the heat and beat in the honey and 2 tbsp of the herbal decoction or rosewater. Add the essential oil, if using.
5 Cool, stirring frequently.
6 Transfer the cream to a sterilised pot or jar. Cover when completely cold. Use within two months.

ELDERFLOWER SKIN NOURISHER Ⓓ

In texture this is like a thick lotion rather than a cream, and spreads very easily over the skin.

3 tbsp dried or 3 heads fresh elderflowers

125 ml (4 fl oz) almond, olive or safflower oil

2 tbsp lanolin

1 Place all the ingredients in the top of a double boiler or in a bowl set in a saucepan of water. Let the lanolin and oil melt together, then keep on a very low heat for 30 minutes.
2 Strain the cream into a small, sterilised pot or jar. Cover when completely cold.

ELDERFLOWER (*Sambucus nigra*)

The elder tree grows in woods, on abandoned land, and often near walls of old or derelict cottages throughout Europe. There are two related species in North America: the American or sweet elder (*Sambucus canadensis*), which is sometimes called elderblow, and the blue berried elder (*Sambucus glauca*), which is cultivated as an ornamental plant along the Pacific coast. Two further species, cultivated mainly for their foliage, are grown in Australia and New Zealand: *Sambucus nigra* and *S. racemosa*.

The creamy-white flower heads of all these trees can be used for cosmetic purposes. Infusions or decoctions of elderflower have a soothing and emollient effect on the skin, and are suitable for all skin types.

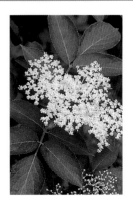

CUCUMBER MOISTURISER Ⓐ

This is good for all skin types. It is a nice green colour and feels very soothing and refreshing when patted onto the skin.

10 cm (4 in) piece cucumber

100 ml (3 fl oz) rosewater

3 tbsp glycerine

1 Finely chop or blend the cucumber, then press it in a sieve to extract the juice.
2 Place the juice, rosewater and glycerine into a sterilised bottle, cover and shake together.
3 Store in a refrigerator and use within one week. Shake well before using.

MARIGOLD MOISTURISER Ⓝ Ⓓ

Use this rich lotion for normal to dry skin and for skin that has been exposed to the sun or wind. The oils will separate from the liquid, but a quick, vigorous shake before use will amalgamate the lotion for a short time.

2 tbsp dried marigolds or 6 fresh marigold heads

150 ml (5 fl oz) water

1 tsp cocoa butter

1 tsp lanolin

4 tbsp sesame or olive oil

1 Place the marigold in a saucepan with the water and bring to the boil. Cover and simmer for ten minutes. Strain off the decoction.
2 Place the cocoa butter, lanolin and oil in the top of a double boiler or in a bowl set in a saucepan of water. Melt them together.
3 Remove entirely from the heat then gradually beat in the marigold infusion. Leave until cold.
4 Transfer the lotion to a sterilised bottle and shake well. Use within six weeks. Shake before use.

ROSEWATER MOISTURISER Ⓐ

This is rich and refreshing at the same time. Like the marigold lotion, the oils will separate, so the lotion will always need a quick shake before use.

1 tsp cocoa butter

1 tsp lanolin

4 tbsp sesame or olive oil

100 ml (3 fl oz) rosewater

2 tbsp witch hazel

1 Place the cocoa butter, lanolin and oil in the top of a double boiler or in a bowl set in a saucepan of water. Melt them together.
2 Gradually beat in the rosewater.
3 Remove entirely from the heat and stir in the witch hazel. Leave until cold.
4 Transfer the lotion to a sterilised bottle and shake well. Use within six weeks. Shake before use.

OILY SKIN MOISTURISER Ⓞ

Oily skin needs a moisturiser that will not add to its oiliness. Yarrow, sage and tincture of benzoin are efficient astringents, and the glycerine provides all the lubrication required.

1 tsp dried or 1 tbsp fresh chopped yarrow or sage

150 ml (5 fl oz) water

100 ml (3 fl oz) rosewater

2 tbsp glycerine

1 tbsp witch hazel

½ tsp tincture of benzoin

1 Place the herb in a saucepan with the water and bring to the boil. Cover and simmer for ten minutes. Cool and strain.
2 Transfer the herbal decoction to a sterilised bottle or jar and add the remaining ingredients. Cover and shake well. Use within two months. Shake well before use.

YARROW (*Achillea millefolium*)

Yarrow grows wild in Europe and throughout North America. In Australia, it is found in cultivation, but it frequently escapes and is considered a troublesome lawn weed. Meadows, pastures, grassy slopes and garden edges are all common habitats for the yarrow plant. It can also be successfully grown in flower and herb gardens.

Yarrow has long stems, feathery leaves that grow in pairs and heads of white flowers that sometimes have a tinge of pink. Its scent is fresh and astringent. Its flowering time is in late summer and it is best cut and dried just as soon as the flower buds open.

SOLVING SKIN PROBLEMS

There are a few skin problems from which most of us suffer at one time or another that can be successfully treated with natural methods.

Spots, blemishes and blackheads

In the teenage years, and sometimes in the years after for those with oily skin, the main problems are spots, blemishes and blackheads. At puberty, hormones run riot and the imbalance often causes extra sebum to be produced. This causes a build-up in the pores. At first the sebum is white.

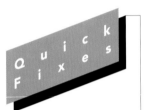

After about eight hours it hardens, is oxidised by the air and then becomes a dreaded blackhead.

If the sebum does not come up to the surface it can form a reddened bump under the skin; this is what we call a blemish. If the skin is not cleansed properly, this bump can turn into a rather nasty pus-filled spot. If you have a lot of spots, then it's acne. This can happen to boys and girls. Girls are most prone just before menstruation when oestrogen production is low. Boys experience the condition when they have a rush of male hormones at puberty.

There are, however, some simple ways to counteract the problem. The first thing is always to cleanse the face thoroughly. Use one of the cleansers recommended for oily skins on pages 27-30. If you use soap, use one that is non-alkaline. The medicated soaps sold with the specific purpose of getting rid of spots may have a sensitising effect on your skin and are not recommended. Try to avoid touching your face during the day, especially if you have spots, because you may spread the infection.

Watch your diet. Avoid processed foods, which are often high in salt and sugar, and low on nutrients. Go easy on the tea and coffee. Eat plenty of fresh fruits and vegetables and high-fibre carbohydrate foods such as brown rice and pasta. Drink plenty of water to cleanse your system.

To get rid of blackheads, steam your face once a week with any of the herbs recommended for oily skin. Steaming softens blackheads, making it easier to remove them with a cotton wool ball. Don't force them or dig in your fingernails. You may make things worse.

Another remedy for blackheads is to give your face a warm oil treatment. It might sound

• If you have wrinkles, use rich moisture creams that contain vitamins E and A, and use toners made from chamomile, linden flowers or lemon balm.

• Try a face mask made of 1 egg yolk beaten with 2 tbsp milk; or any mask that contains lanolin or mashed bananas.

odd, treating oil with oil, but it again has a softening effect. Have ready a face cloth and a bowl of hot water. Massage a little almond or olive oil into your face. Wring the face cloth out in the hot water and lay it over the affected areas. Let it become cool, wring it out, and lay it on again. Do this several more times until the water begins to get cool. Once again, push out the blackheads with a cotton wool ball.

Wrinkles and threadveins

Wrinkles are a 'problem' that affect us all in the end. The secret is to think about wrinkles early and keep them at bay for as long as possible. Besides following the cleanse, tone and moisturise routine, take care of your diet and keep your facial muscles in tone.

Many a time when we were children, we were told that if we made an awful face and the wind blew, our face would stay in that position. It was just a threat to make us behave, but there is more truth in it than you would think. Wrinkles are caused by our continually making the same expression. This causes the same facial muscles to contract all the time and they eventually become permanently shortened. The skin cannot contract like the muscle, so a dip appears in it which becomes a wrinkle.

It is fascinating to look at children's faces. Unless they are unusually ill or disturbed, their faces are smooth and unlined, and they often look similar to each other. After puberty, we pull faces to match how we think and feel and our characters and experiences become etched on our faces.

We don't, however, want our experiences to show that much. So we should remember to relax our faces as often as possible. Facial exercises and massage may help to reduce wrinkles, and prevent more from developing. Regular use of nourishing and exfoliating face masks will also help to keep your skin soft. (See page 33 for how to apply a face mask.)

Excessive exposure to extremes of weather can cause dry or chapped skin, which in turn leads to wrinkling. Always use a sunblock when you are outside, and moisturise your skin well. (See The Effects of the Sun, page 93.)

Threadveins are tiny, broken blood vessels that are visible through the skin, particularly on the face. Drinking too much alcohol can encourage the production of threadveins by depriving the body of B vitamins. Washing with water that is too hot can also lead to the formation of threadveins on delicate facial skin. If you have threadveins, never steam your face.

CUCUMBER AND GLYCERINE HAND LOTION Ⓐ

Like all glycerine hand lotions, this one isn't greasy. The cucumber makes it very moisturising.

one 2.5 cm (1 in) piece cucumber

2 tbsp glycerine

2 tbsp rosewater

2 tbsp vodka or brandy

1 Peel, finely chop and mash the cucumber in a bowl.
2 Add the remaining ingredients to the cucumber pulp.
3 Transfer to a sterilised pot or jar and store in a refrigerator. Use within one week.

CONDITIONING MASSAGE CREAM Ⓐ

Use this massage cream once a week to keep your hands soft and smooth. The almonds and oatmeal slough off dead skin cells, and the herbal infusion is soothing. If you don't have ground almonds, add an extra teaspoon of oatmeal.

1 tsp dried lady's mantle, elderflowers or marigolds

100 ml (3 fl oz) boiling water

1 tbsp fine oatmeal

1 tsp ground almonds

1 tsp almond, avocado or olive oil

1 tsp glycerine

1 tsp lemon juice

1 Place the herb into a sterilised jug or bowl. Pour on the boiling water, cover and leave until cold. Strain.
2 Place the oatmeal and ground almonds in a bowl and mix in the oil, glycerine, lemon juice and 1 tbsp of the herbal infusion. Use immediately.
3 Massage the mixture into your hands. After massaging, leave the mixture on for 20 minutes.
4 Rinse off with tepid water and apply a hand cream if wished.

LEMON AND LADY'S MANTLE HAND LOTION Ⓝ Ⓞ

This light, non-greasy lotion both softens and whitens the hands. Lavender, marigold flowers or elderflowers can be used instead of the lady's mantle to make the herbal decoction. Alternatively, use rosewater.

1 tsp dried or 1 tbsp fresh chopped lady's mantle

150 ml (5 fl oz) water

4 tbsp lemon juice

4 tbsp glycerine

2 tbsp vodka

1 Place the lady's mantle and water in a saucepan and bring to the boil. Simmer for five minutes. Cool and strain.
2 Pour 4 tbsp of the decoction into a sterilised bottle. Add the other ingredients and shake well. Store in a refrigerator and use within one week.
3 Apply daily to your hands, massaging it in well. Shake before use.

LADY'S MANTLE (*Alchemilla vulgaris*)

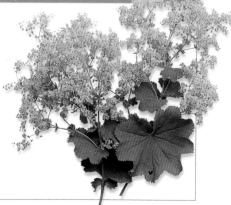

Lady's mantle is a herb that has been used mainly for menstrual disorders, but which also has soothing and wound-healing properties. It is an attractive herb with large, circular leaves, rather like fans, and branches of small yellow flowers. In the herb garden it grows to the height of about 50 cm (20 in) and likes a moist soil.

RECIPE — TREATMENT FOR CHAPPED HANDS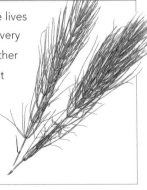

Warm milk is a soothing treatment for chapped hands. Make up a simple, rich cream to use afterwards.

For the cream:

3 tbsp lanolin

1 tbsp olive oil

one 250 iu vitamin E capsule (optional)

For the treatment:

300 ml (10 fl oz) whole milk

2 hand-sized pieces cotton wool

1 Place the lanolin and olive oil in the top of a double boiler or in a bowl set in a saucepan of water. Melt them together on a low heat, stirring frequently.
2 Prick the vitamin E capsule and squeeze the contents into the saucepan.
3 Remove the cream from the heat and cool it, beating frequently.
4 Transfer the cream to a sterilised pot or jar. Cover when completely cold and use within one month.
5 Pour the warmed milk into a bowl. Soak the cotton wool pieces in the milk. Lay one on each hand. Keep them there for 20 minutes. Massage any moisture left on your hands into the skin.
6 Massage in some of the cream.

RECIPE — NAIL-CONDITIONING MASSAGE CREAM

Massage this into your nails every day for a week and they will become healthy and strong. After that, use once a week to maintain the effect.

1 egg yolk

2 tbsp almond, avocado or olive oil

1 tsp honey

¼ tsp sea salt

1 Place the egg yolk in a bowl and beat in the oil, honey and salt.
2 Use immediately, massaging the mixture into your nails, taking about five minutes for each hand. Do not wash off the residue until the following morning.

RECIPE — NAIL-STRENGTHENING CREAM

Horsetail is a renowned nail strengthener. Massage this cream into your fingernails daily.

1 tbsp dried or 2 tbsp fresh chopped horsetail

4 tbsp boiling water

1 tbsp cocoa butter

1 tbsp lanolin

1 Place the horsetail in a bowl and pour on the boiling water. Cover and leave until cold. Strain.
2 Place the cocoa butter and lanolin in the top of a double boiler or in a bowl set in a saucepan of water. Melt them gently together on a low heat.
3 Beat in 1 tbsp of the horsetail infusion.
4 Remove entirely from the heat and beat until the cream has cooled.
5 Transfer the cream to a sterilised pot. Cover when completely cold and use within two months.

HORSETAIL (*Equisetum arvense*)

Horsetail is a spectacular plant that in appearance lives up to its folk name of bottlebrush. It is tall, with very thin, spiky leaves that make it look like a brush or feather duster. In prehistoric times it grew as tall as a tree, but today it can be found up to 1 metre (3 feet) high. Horsetail is rich in silica, making it an excellent external treatment for broken or weak nails.

Horsetail is toxic in large doses and should never be taken internally.

MANICURE

Manicured nails greatly enhance the look of your hands. Try to find time once a week for a treatment.

What you will need:

cotton wool balls

emery board

150 ml (5 fl oz) warm water or infusion of horsetail

bowl

4 tbsp sunflower, olive or almond oil

cotton buds

towel

nail buffer, soft cloth or piece of chamois leather

hand cream or lotion

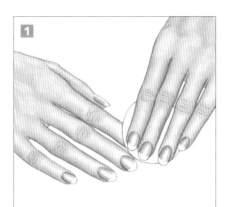

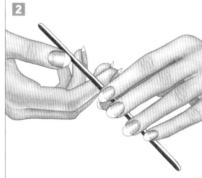

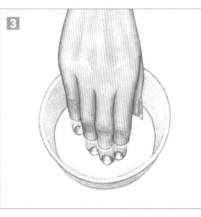

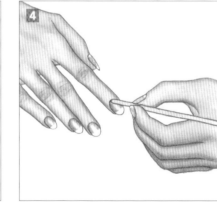

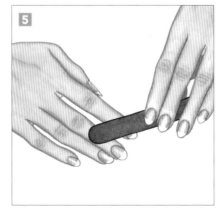

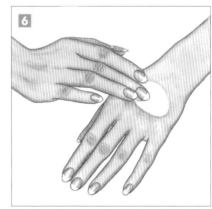

1 Remove any nail polish.
2 Shape the nails with an emery board, not a metal nail file. Work in one direction only and do not take them too far down at the corners. Aim for almond-shaped or squared nails.
3 Pour the warm water or infusion into a bowl. Add the oil. Dabble your fingertips in this for ten minutes. Dry gently.
4 Using a cotton bud, gently press back the cuticles. (They should never be cut.)
5 Buff your nails.
6 Massage in hand cream or lotion.

F E E T

soothe

invigorate

moisturise

exercise

massage

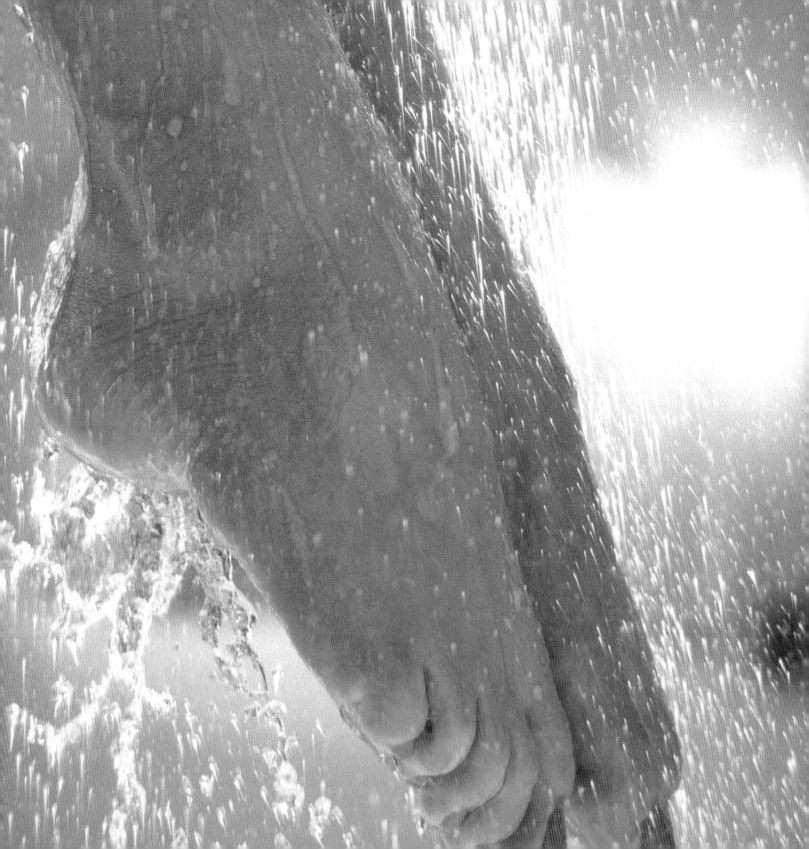

Your feet and legs support you throughout the day, helping you to walk, run, climb and dance, so give them some attention. Feet have to take the weight of your whole body, and in order to do this efficiently, they need to spread out naturally. It pays, therefore, to buy well-fitting shoes that give you a certain amount of support. If you have normal or narrow feet, this will be relatively easy. If you have wide feet, you may have to look further.

We humans were not designed to walk on our toes: high heels make us lean forwards and stick out our bottoms at an awkward angle. By all means wear high heels for special occasions and when you want to feel elegant, but choose something flatter for every day.

Encasing your feet in tights or stockings also constricts the toes, so kick off your shoes, take off the nylons, and walk barefoot whenever you can. Wriggle your toes occasionally to keep them supple.

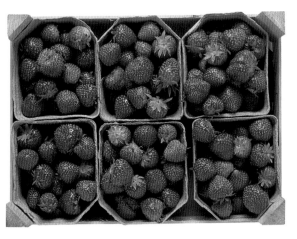

Activities that help to keep legs and feet in shape include swimming, cycling, walking, yoga or stretching exercises

Legs have fewer sebaceous glands than any other part of the body, and the calves are often the place where uncared-for skin begins to look dry and flaky. So, whenever you moisturise your body, pay particular attention to your legs, especially if you have been out in the sun.

Exfoliate your legs with the 'Salt and oil body rub' (see page 89) or by rubbing with a pumice stone, loofah or hand mitt when you are in the bath. If your knees look dry and flaky, use the 'Elbow softener' treatment given on page 89.

Footbaths

If you feel brave and are in need of a good body toner or early morning reviver, try a cold footbath. Fill a plastic bowl with enough cold water to cover your ankles. With a plastic beaker, pour the water over your calves. Then

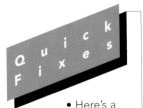

Quick Fixes

• Here's a simple booster for tired legs and feet: lie down with your feet above your head for ten minutes. Then, with a light coating of oil on your hands, gently massage each leg in turn with continual movements from ankle to knee.

quickly towel yourself dry. You can also hold the shower nozzle and sit with just your feet in the stream of cold water.

Herbal footbaths revive and relieve aching feet, and make the rest of the body feel good, too. The skin on your feet is surprisingly absorbent. To try this out, rub a small amount of peppermint oil on your soles. Within about twenty minutes you will begin to taste peppermint. With this in mind, add herbs to your footbath that suit your needs. For a list, see 'Herbs to add to your bath' on pages 78-79. Dried herbs should be tied in a piece of muslin or cotton. Fresh herbs can be used on the sprig. This will prevent too much mess. For the method, see the recipes below.

After any kind of bath, always dry your feet well, especially between the toes, to prevent infections such as athlete's foot.

SOLVING PROBLEMS

Corns form as a protection against tight shoes or constant rubbing, so in addition to treating the corn try to sort out the cause. Small corns can usually be dealt with by using a pumice stone when you use a footbath or have a bath. You can also try the garlic treatment. Rub the corn with a cut clove of garlic, then take one sliver of garlic and secure it onto the corn with plaster or a bandage. Replace it daily until the corn disappears. If this doesn't work, consult a chiropodist.

If you suffer from smelly feet, take a daily footbath made with deodorising herbs such as basil or lovage, and dry and powder your feet well afterwards.

FOOT MASSAGE

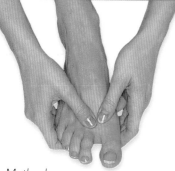

Use a base oil such as almond, avocado, jojoba or wheatgerm. Choose either refreshing or relaxing essential oils to add to it.

What you will need:
towel
base oil

Method:
1 Rest your feet on a towel. Coat your hands and feet in a thin film of oil.
2 Place both hands either side of one foot, with your thumbs on top and all fingers underneath. Place your thumbs in the centre of your foot and gradually draw them outwards to the sides of the foot. Do this six times.
3 With your hands in the same position, massage the tops of your foot with small circular movements of your thumbs.
4 Turn your foot over and rest it on your other leg. Place your hands in the same position, but this time with your thumbs on the soles of your feet. Massage with the same circular movements.
5 Press your thumbs firmly all over the sole of your foot.
6 Hold each toe in turn with your thumb in front and your forefinger underneath. Gently squeeze the toe and give it a firm tug.
7 With your foot upright, hold it with a hand on either side. Stroke with long, slow movements from toe to ankle.

REFRESHING HERBAL FOOTBATH

This will relax and refresh tired feet and legs.

1 tsp dried or 1 tbsp fresh rosemary

1 tsp dried or 1 tbsp fresh peppermint

2 tbsp sea salt

enough boiling water to fill bowl

juice ½ lemon

1 Place the herbs in the bowl and add the sea salt.
2 Pour enough boiling water into the bowl to cover your feet.
3 Lay a large towel over the bowl and leave until the water has cooled down sufficiently for you to put your feet into it.
4 Add the lemon juice.
5 Soak your feet in the footbath for as long as you wish, but don't let the water get cold.

HERBAL FOOTBATH TO SOOTHE SORE FEET

Use this after a hard day on your feet.

1 tsp dried or 1 tbsp fresh lavender flowers

1 tbsp dried elderflowers or 2 fresh elderflower heads

1 tbsp dried chamomile or 6 fresh chamomile flowers

enough boiling water to fill bowl

1 Place the herbs in the bowl.
2 Pour enough boiling water into the bowl to cover your feet.
3 Lay a large towel over the bowl and leave until the water has cooled down sufficiently for you to put your feet into it.
4 Soak your feet in the footbath for as long as you wish, but don't let the water get cold.

COMFORTING HERBAL FOOTBATH

This is a footbath to relax both your feet and your spirits.

1 tsp dried or 1 tbsp fresh lavender flowers

1 tsp dried or 1 tbsp fresh comfrey leaves

8 scented geranium leaves, if available

1 tbsp Epsom salts or washing soda

enough boiling water to fill bowl

1 Place the herbs and the other ingredients in the bowl.
2 Pour enough boiling water into the bowl to cover your feet.
3 Lay a large towel over the bowl and leave until the water has cooled down sufficiently for you to put your feet into it.
4 Soak your feet in the footbath for as long as you wish, but don't let the water get cold.

SCENTED GERANIUM LEAVES

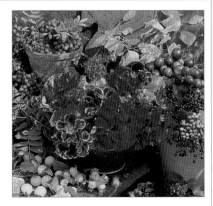

What are often referred to as scented geraniums are in fact pelargoniums, whose beauty is in the shape and fragrance of their leaves. Some are soft and furry, others ridged and deeply cut; their scents range from fresh mints and lemons to the sweet and resinous.

You can grow scented geraniums in pots, keep them for years, and take cuttings regularly to ensure that you have a good supply of leaves. Keep them indoors in winter and outdoors in summer. Water them regularly, feed in summer and cut them back twice a year to keep them healthy and bushy.

Scented geraniums can sometimes be picked up quite cheaply at summer fairs and street markets. Otherwise, go to a specialist nursery or a herb grower. You need your own supplies as geranium leaves are seldom available dried.